C000139864

SELF-MASSAGE
Secrets

A Short Guidebook to Self-Healing Through Massage

NIKO CARRAFIELD

WHAT PEOPLE ARE SAYING
ABOUT NIKO'S CLINIC

"Chi Nei Tsang is an extensive abdominal massage that clears the deepest of energies. I felt for the first time ever, I was able to see inside myself, and I was being given access to heal."

–Lou C, *Patient*

"Niko helped me with (L5) Sciatic Nerve pain in my lower back, pelvis, rotator cup/shoulder, quads, and knees hurt too. I've had this pain in my body for 13 years and was told I needed to get surgery and pre-scribed pharmaceutical drugs with expenses costing $7k.

In just the first session I started to feel relief of stress, anxiety, and depression after so many years. My body started to feel rejuvenated healing my organs and re-lieving my nervous system. I feel clear now and I highly suggest everyone experience "Chi Nei Tsang". I can fi-nally relax and not suffer anymore thanks to this ther-apy!"

–Danny Z, *Patient*

"I appreciate how detailed and thorough Niko is in explaining what is being done through the entire pro-cess. I have shared with friends and family to go see him for their ailments and look forward to going back again to see him on a regular basis to keep myself feel-ing better physically and mentally."

–Carolyn C, *Patient*

AUTHOR'S NOTE

In this book, we will be focusing on the main points of the body for relaxing and restoring the nervous system and improving circulation. You can perform these techniques while lying down, sitting or standing at any time.

These techniques are not meant to replace or substitute for a medical doctor so please talk with your physician before, during, and after the reading and practicing of this material.

Thank you for your time and attention, and may this book serve you as well as the information and experience have served me.

DEDICATION

This book is dedicated to my mother, Diana, for first introducing acupressure and healing through massage into my life.

I'd like to thank God for my mother's guidance, discipline, and devotion to the teachings of Jesus Christ. Praise God and the highest powers of healing and grace.

Self-Massage Secrets
Copyright © 2020 Niko Carrafield.

All rights reserved. No part of this publication may be reproduced, stored in a retrieval system, or transmitted, in any form or by any means, electronic, mechanical, photocopying, recording or otherwise, without the prior permission of the publishers.

The author asserts the moral right to be identified as the author of this work.

First Edition, 2020

Visit **NewLifeCNT.com** for bulk book purchases and curriculum.

Book design by Bethany Guajardo using Adobe® InDesign.® Set in Brandon Grotesque for the header, Gotham for the body text and Bebas Neue for the chapter titles and headers • TeamBeth.com

TABLE OF CONTENTS

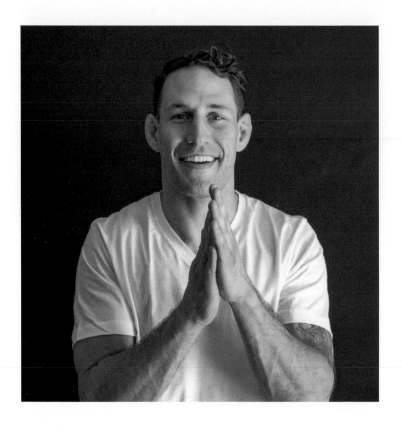

INTRODUCTION

LEARN HOW TO RELIEVE STRESS AND PAIN BY BALANCING ENERGY

This short book is intended as a daily instructional checklist designed to take you through the main keys needed to release chronic pain, balance energy, and reduce overall stress. The unique philosophy guiding this specific type of self-massage is derived from the ancient practice of **Chi Nei Tsang**, a Traditional Chinese Medicine. The body holds tension accumulated from chronic mental, emotional, and physical stress which can shift posture and create misalignment, the root cause of unnecessary pain.

When nerves, arteries, and veins become blocked they prevent the healing process. By opening these channels through conscious massage, breathing, and meditation you can realign and restore proper communication and circulation within the body.

You may read each technique and practice along as you read, or, after reading each section, pause, put down the book, and take 1-2 minutes for each instruction while breathing and focusing on its effect. Take the time to feel each point before moving on, connecting your mind to the body and remembering each point intentionally for more lasting results.

By releasing and relaxing each point one by one, you will experience a more sustained relaxation and overall control of the nervous system, switching from sympathetic (fight or flight) to parasympathetic (rest and digest), simply by being aware and using these techniques.

If you want to view each exercise in further detail, visit **Academy.NewLifeCNT.com** and watch the video course.

KEY THINGS TO REMEMBER

Set an Intention

It is vital to keep a positive outlook while massaging, tapping, or hitting the body because you are affecting the subconscious mind within every cell of your body. Focus and hold the intention of positive energy and healing. Knowing and imagining each cell is reproducing youthful and healthy cells as you massage, relax, and restore.

Deep Breathing

It is essential to be aware of your breath while doing these exercises and acupressure.Inhaling new **prana, Chi,** or **life-force energy** with each breath. Then exhaling stale Chi, toxins, or bad energy out. The amazing and invisible magic of intention, combined with the breath, allows you to release mental and physical elements with each exhale.

Burping/Yawning

Burping and yawning are helpful for releasing stuck energy and opening the body for fresh blood and Chi. Burping is useful for eliminating trapped gas that can transform into sick energy if not released. Yawning is beneficial because of its ability to stretch the inner body, stretching deep layers of fascia and moving Chi.

TYPES OF TOUCH

There are multiple types of touch to get the precise effect. Using the right amount of pressure for the right amount of time is important to open each channel and organ, healing nervous tension. Use the following techniques for each of the various points, taking time to feel the effects in your own body.

Thumb

The thumb can be a tool for holding pressure for a longer duration and useful when gripping with the index and middle finger or all four fingers. Use the tip or the edge of the thumb in places like the chin, jaw, eye socket, and in-between joints like the knees, elbows, forearms, and wrists. The base of the thumb is better used to squeeze places like the neck, inner arms, hips or iliac bone, thighs, calves, and inner arches.

Index and Middle Finger

The index finger and middle fingers can be used individually, together, or along with the thumb to squeeze particular areas of the body. The pressure from these fingers is lighter and in the case of a very sensitive spot, used to warm a point before using the thumb, knuckles, or elbow for a deeper massage. Both the index finger and middle finger can be applied in places like the eyes, nose, ears, across the collarbone, into the ribs, the sternum, and getting into smaller areas of the organs.

Four Fingers

You can use the four fingers for the belly and abdomen to pulsate, circle, and open space for blood and Chi to flow in and out of the organs.

With the four fingers together, form a "C" shape with the hand. Use the tip of the fingers to dig under the rib cage on either side where the liver, gallbladder, stomach, and spleen are located (read the following sections labeled for each organ for more explanation). Make a scooping motion to open space for the organs to flow and function better, releasing tension while breathing deeply into the abdomen.

Elbow

The elbows are an invaluable tool for massaging the limbs. Using the elbows on the forearms and hands is best, as each hand may not be able to give enough pressure or go deep enough to find the relief. When using the elbows on the forearms, be sure to bring the forearm to the elbow. The elbows also work wonders on the thighs, calves, and feet.

Fist and Knuckles

Using the knuckles can offer a more solid way of holding pressure rather than using the thumb or four fingers. For example, massaging the temples with the thumbs can work well and allow for the release you need, however, the knuckles can be used for a deeper hold without exhausting the thumb. Also, the knuckles are great for the hips, low back, and kidneys when you're not able to use an elbow or get enough pressure from using the fingers or thumbs.

Palm

The palm or open hand is used to calm, cool, or heat an area while also circling and moving Chi. When applying the palms on the body, start with gentle pressure, gradually increasing compression from light to a firm squeeze. The palms can be used for massaging the temples, front and back of the skull, both sides of the neck or squeezing both sides of either knee.

The palms can also help to stabilize, charge, or detoxify Chi. A simple squeeze of the joints, brain, and arteries helps to release stagnant energy trapped in the head, chest, or abdomen. Squeezing both sides of the carotid arteries of the neck can help to balance the blood to either side of the brain relieving headaches and other sensory disorders. The palms can also be used to alleviate pain in the knee, hip, or ankle.

CLEANSING BREATH

A cleansing breath happens when you inhale through your nose and exhale through your mouth. When you inhale through your nose, prana, Chi or lifeforce energy passes through the brain allowing you to direct the energy anywhere in your body.

- Inhale deeply through the nose for 3-5 seconds.
- Retain for 1-3 seconds.
- Exhale through the mouth with a sigh.
- Sustain at the end of your breath for 1-3 seconds.
- Relax more with each exhale and repeat.

HITTING

After each massage, lightly hitting the muscles and tendons of the body can benefit the nervous system, blood, and Chi. By tapping, knocking, hitting or pounding the body and bones you are effectively energizing the blood, fascia, and Chi. The blood can flow, flush and transform better, strengthening it on a cellular level.

With intention, this doubles the impact of the meditation or mantra being used. After massaging and meditating you may hit the body all over or specifically as you wish, to instill intention and prayer into your flesh and cells reproducing healthier blood and fresh Chi into the bones and tendons.

- As you complete your massage make a fist and or use your palms to gently hit the bones of the feet and ankles to strengthen the ankles and shin bones.
- Follow up by hitting the knees, thighs, and hips. Strike the whole body, abdomen, rib cage, arms, neck, and even the head to stabilize the bones of the entire body and stimulate Chi circulation.

FEEL THE CHI

In **reflexology**, the hands hold the connection to the rest of the body and rubbing them together is very good for the nervous system.

- Begin by rubbing the hands together until warm (approximately 1-2 minutes).
- Rub the hands front and back vigorously to create heat.
- Hold the hands 2-3 inches apart and feel the warmth.
- Hover the hands over the face and feel the warmth and Chi behind your eyes.

QIGONG BREATHING

Standing after your massage and breathing

into the entire body is important for opening and activating blood, muscles and energetic channels. To do this:

- Stand up and firmly plant both feet on the ground, inhale lifting both arms, palms up, out to the sides, and above your head.
- At the same time, come up on your toes to activate and pull energy up from the feet to the kidneys by squeezing the buttocks and pelvis, then pulling the diaphragm up and into the heart, and tucking the chin into the head.
- Exhale and bring the hands and heels down slowly, palms down with thumbs pointed inward.
- Repeat this 3-6 times after your massage to increase Chi flow and balance energy.

To see each exercise in detail on video, please visit **Academy.NewLifeCNT.com** *and watch the course.*

THIS PAGE IS
INTENTIONALLY LEFT BLANK

PART I

UPPER BODY

WHAT IS SHEN?

According to Traditional Chinese Medicine theory, **"Shen"** is one of the three "treasures" or larger energies we have as human beings. *Shen* is **"our spirit, conscious mind and our universal connection."** In other words, it's our thoughts. *Shen* derives from *Chi* (heart force) and *Jing* (sexual energy), and yet overall *Shen,* influences and energizes both. The goal is to clarify, condense and concentrate these three major energy groups in unison to find enlightenment (the lightened path or flow).

In dealing with common upper body issues like the ones listed below, we must first understand that we are the energy we allow ourselves to produce and work with. Relaxing the mind, the body, and our emotions starts with *Shen*, the thought and motivation to find ease. Follow through the instructions below with a positive and healing intention, clearing and cleansing the body and the brain's energetic field.

COMMON UPPER BODY ISSUES

Common upper body issues include but are not limited to; headaches, migraines, eye pain or strains, tinnitus, neck pain and strains, cramps, TMJ or grinding of the teeth, colds and bacterial infections, as well as acne and other skin disorders.

EYES

The eyes are responsible for receiving a large amount of information. When we have habits of staring for too long, especially at screens with blue light, the eyes tense up from overactivity. Like tendonitis, overuse can cause pain in various parts of the connecting tendons.

The brain, surrounding senses, neck, shoulders, hands, and the rest of the body can be affected by the eyes. Relaxing the tendons behind the eyes can benefit the body and brain in numerous ways, improving vision and the nervous system.

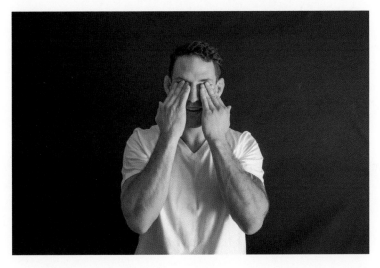

- Start by lightly pressing both palms into the

eyes, holding for 1-3 cleansing breaths. This will help to relax the muscles and tendons before massaging.

- Lightly massage around the eyes, pressing into the bones of the face, the eyebrows, bridge of the nose, and top of the cheekbone under the eyes.
- Stretch the tendons behind the eyes by pressing the fingers lightly into the space between the eye and the upper and lower bone of the eye socket.
- With the eyelids closed use both thumbs to press into the bottom of the eyebrows just above the eyelids.
- Press the thumb into the space behind the eyeball, stretching the tendons behind the eyes.
- Relax the hands and with eyes still closed, look up...down...left...right...and circle the eyes both clockwise and counterclockwise slowly 3-6x.
- Inhale deeply through the nose while gently pulling up on the pelvic floor and breathing intentionally into the eyes, imagining new blood and oxygen flowing in and around the eyes.

TEMPLES

The tissue here on either side of the forehead and skull can block energy along the frontal lobe of the brain. Clearing the temples of tension can help to prevent headaches, eye, ear, and sinus issues. By massaging the temples regularly you are telling the subconscious mind and frontal lobe to relax, helping you to focus and find clarity.

- Use both thumbs simultaneously and press

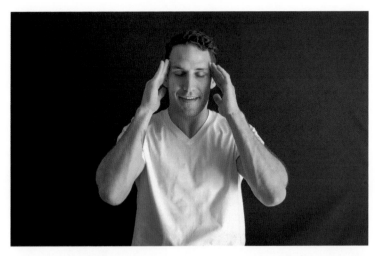

into the temples slowly. Hold, circle and slide the thumbs back alongside the temples toward the back of the ears.

- Take 3-5 deep cleansing breaths while continuing to hold, pushing, pressing and massaging in circular motions to release tension.
- Feel, breathe deeply, and release any large knots. Releasing these knots can help to prevent headaches and colds.
- Next, squeeze both palms to either side of the temples simultaneously, making small, slow circles in an up and down motion.
- While applying pressure with the palms use the fingers to massage the top of the head into the scalp and top of the skull.
- This helps release tension and stimulates hair follicles.
- Finally, make a fist with both hands and rub the index knuckles into each side of the temples, holding and breathing as necessary for efficient release.

OCCIPUT

The occiput is located at the back of the skull. This particular area can hold tension often accumulated from poor posture. When stress builds within the body, signals are sent to the brain through the spinal cord. This can cause knots to form along the back of the neck, skull, and spine. These knots disrupt communication between nerves which can lead to headaches and chronic pain.

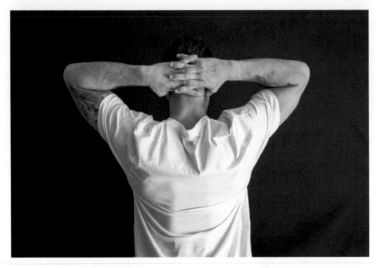

- Interlace both hands together behind the head and with both thumbs, begin pressing, massaging and squeezing both sides of the cervical spine.
- Below and along the lining of the back of the skull, massage from the middle to the bones behind the ears.
- With the thumbs, keep pressure just below the bone behind the ears.
- Now, move the thumbs back and forth to

loosen and release tension between the skull and the spine.

- As you clear pain and tension away from this area it will open channels and connections to the eyes, ears, and senses and help relieve and prevent headaches.

EARS

Massaging the ears regularly will restore energy throughout the body. This is because the kidneys and ears are connected along similar meridian channels. Tension from each organ builds and stores within the face and ears. By rubbing the ears daily you will energetically soothe the body.

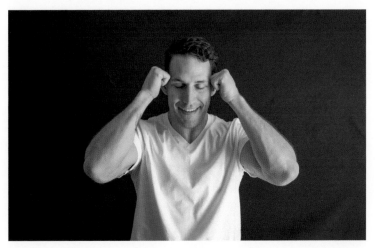

- Press into the **tragus** (the little triangle-shaped cartilage that sticks out in front of the ear) with the index finger, holding and releasing quickly.
- Next, wiggle the index finger inside the ear canal lightly, popping the fingers out to shake and open the ear canal.
- Massage the back of the ears where you feel

the skull and ear meet.

- Fold the ear forward, hold and release for 10-30 seconds.
- Finally, use your index finger and thumb to rub the entire ear until warm, approximately 30-60 seconds.

JAW

The heart directly affects the tension of the jaw for multiple reasons. The heart is the closest to the jaw connected by the **SCM** (*sternocleidomastoid muscle*) or front neck muscles. When the jaw becomes tight from forward head posture, slumping, texting, driving, and or computers, the heart and jaw tighten energetically. When matters of the heart are not expressed the jaw clenches. Opening the mouth, hitting the jaw and teeth, and massaging the front neck and chin will help to open the heart and relieve tension in the jaw.

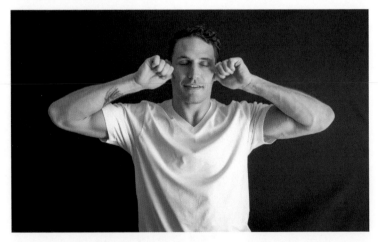

- Start by using the thumbs to simultaneously apply pressure to either side of the jaw.

- Once pressure is applied, massage in small circular motions, pressing into the cheek or jawbones where the back molars are located, just in front of the ears.
- Use the thumb, index and middle fingers to squeeze the lining of the jaw (mandible or chin).
- Massage down the lining of the jaw, starting from the ear to the tip of the chin.
- There may be knots or "masses" underneath the chin, so be sure to hold and work out these bumps before or even after they've become hard or bone-like.
- The knuckles can also be used to add additional pressure.
- Finally, press both palms to the side of the jaw simultaneously, making small, slow circles in an up and down motion while opening and closing the jaw.

TEETH AND CHEEKBONES

Massaging the gums and cheekbone is extremely beneficial for the overall health of the mouth. Stress from the heart and underlying organs creates tension affecting the gums and teeth. Regularly massaging and hitting the gums will clear tension and stagnant Chi, allowing for better blood flow and healthier gums to support the teeth.

- Squeeze the tops of the cheekbones with the index and middle fingers while digging into the gums with the thumbs to relieve stress and tension from the teeth.
- Next, tap the four fingers into the cheeks, knocking the teeth 100 times (hitting the

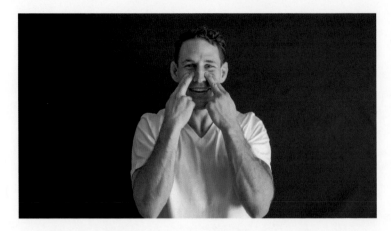

gums on the front, sides, top, and bottom).
- You can also use the knuckles to gently knock the teeth and jaw for more strength.

CHIN

Underneath the chin lies the bottom of the tongue. Over long durations of stress, masses of tissue develop and store toxic Chi. Releasing these knots may take time but massaging the surrounding tissue will help to open up cells to receive new blood and Chi.

- Using your four fingers and thumbs, press into the bones of the chin.
- Massage into the front side of the chin making small circles with your four fingers.
- With the thumbs, dig into the underside of the chin, feeling for bumps, knots, or sensitive areas along the chin bone.
- Continue to massage feeling into the tongue and throat.
- Press and hold at any particular sensitive point for 30-90 seconds, 3-9 breaths.

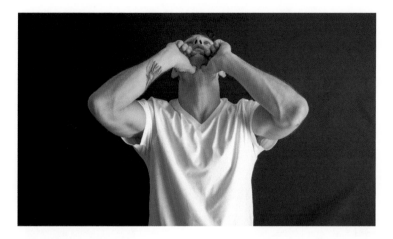

NECK

The neck can hide a lot of emotional tension that comes from various other places in the body. Use the thumbs to apply pressure to the surrounding muscle of the cervical spine. You will re-align the vertebrae over time and help to restructure imbalances. This will help to alleviate headaches, nerve pains, and impingements, as well as prevent and reverse chronic pain.

- Interlace both hands behind the head, then take both thumbs and squeeze each disc of the neck, clearing tension and knots between the small spaces of each vertebra.
- Once pressure is applied, you can begin to oscillate your head side to side in a "no" motion to release tension.
- Follow the length of the neck down to where the shoulders meet and feel for any abnormalities (knots, bumps, one side larger than the other), balancing with the appropriate pressure while shaking your head away from the tension.

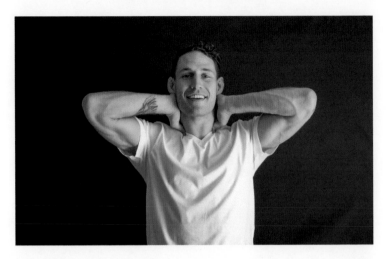

- Squeeze the neck with the palms on either side.
- Hold for 20 seconds and release for 10, breathing deeply and calmly.
- You may feel light-headed while doing this practice, but if you breathe sufficiently and let go when it feels necessary, you should feel the balancing effects and benefits after a few times practicing.

THYROID

The thyroid is an energetic point within the body for control and expression. The thyroid helps the immune system by providing hormones that regulate vital body functions such as breathing, heart rate, central and peripheral nervous systems, body weight, and muscle strength.

- Moving to the front of the neck, grab the throat with each hand, squeezing and massaging both sides of the carotid arteries and SCM muscles.

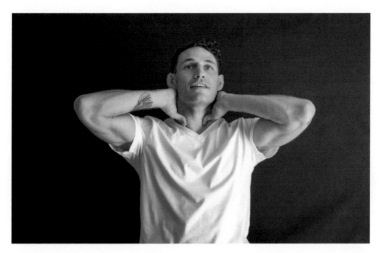

- If you begin to cough, good, it's your body clearing out stale energy and oxygen and bringing in new blood to strengthen the throat and thyroid.
- Hold 30-90 seconds on any point where you feel a knot. Make sure to dig deep into the throat, don't be too gentle, you need to break up the deep muscular tension for proper blood flow and healing.
- Massage out the pain but go at your own pace, it will loosen up over time so do it a little bit every day.

*To see each exercise in detail on video, please visit **Academy.NewLifeCNT.com** and watch the course.*

*THIS PAGE IS
INTENTIONALLY LEFT BLANK*

PART 2

MID-BODY

PART 2
MID-BODY

WHAT IS CHI?

"Chi" [also spelled Qi or Ki] is the Chinese word for *"energy as it relates to bio-electricity."* The electricity in our blood, cells, and the entire body is powered by bio-electricity or *Chi* and gives us the ability to move, breathe, and live. *Chi* is everywhere, in every living thing and with our intention we can develop it, direct it and use it for healing.

With healing in mind, self-massage can soothe and restore good *Chi* within the cells of the body. Follow the instructions below to soothe the heart, making sure to smile, creating positive emotion while breathing fully to open the lungs and energy field for more healing *Chi*.

COMMON MIDDLE BODY ISSUES

Common mid-body issues include but are not limited to; chest pain, heart pain, heartburn, trouble breathing, shoulder tears and impingements, numbing of the hands, tendonitis, arthritis, carpal tunnel, neck strains, headache, back pain, feelings of anxiety, grief or depression, soreness, and other issues.

SHOULDERS

Shoulder pain can derive from rounded shoulders, forward head posture and other postural misalignments, injuries, repetitive movements, nervous tension, and emotional pain. When experiencing a lack of range of motion from an impingement or nerve pain, this may be restored once the tension from the **brachial plexus** is released.

The brachial plexus is found on the front side of the neck just above the collar bone on either side of the throat. Follow the instructions below to relax this area, effectively loosening the nerves connecting to the hands and head.

To massage the shoulder it is best to rest your arm on a table or armrest so that the shoulder is more relaxed and open.

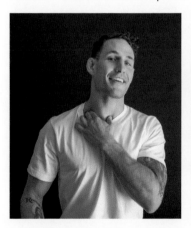 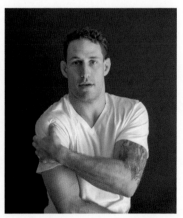

- Start by gripping the shoulder with the four fingers and thumb.
- With the thumb, dig into the front of the shoulder where it meets the chest and clavicle.

- Apply pressure and release quickly or make small half-circles to massage away tension.
- Continue massaging around the chest area to the side of the shoulder.
- Use the index and middle fingers to press and massage into the side of the shoulder where it connects to the humerus bone (upper arm bone).
- Continue using the index and four fingers up and around to the back, massaging into the **trapezius** (traps) muscle going up the back of the neck.
- Apply pressure into the trapezius, massaging the muscle and nerves underneath to release tension in this area.
- Move down and around the neck just above the clavicle to find the brachial plexus (on either side of the neck). To release the tension here, use the index and middle finger to hold pressure.
- Inhale and raise your arm up.
- Exhale and relax your arm down.
- Continue circling your arm while applying pressure into these points.
- By placing pressure here you can loosen the tension to the fingers. You may experience a tingling sensation or numbness in the arm moving down to the tips of the fingers.
- Once you feel this, you must breathe deeply, centering your mind into the fingers.
- Open the fingers and wrists while inhaling, circling the wrists in both directions.
- Lastly, squeeze and massage into the humerus bone entirely, pulling the bicep and

tricep muscles away from the bone. If you find a place where the tissue seems harder than the other areas, use the thumb for added strength.

- Do this until the numbness goes away and shoulder mobility improves.
- Once you finish one arm, do the same for the other arm.

ARMPIT

Prolonged emotional stress from the heart and lungs will affect the armpit blocking the lymph nodes and creating knots. These bundles of distorted tissue harm the surrounding cells over time. Most often the tissue is energetically deprived and within minutes of massage, it will become healthier and more alive than before. Follow the steps included here to loosen and open these lymph nodes and nerves for better flow of fluids and Chi.

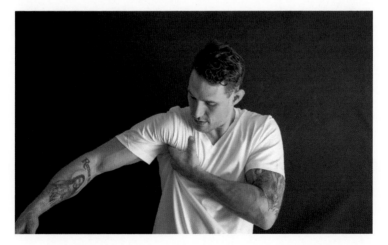

- Start by using the thumb to massage into the armpit.

- Dig the thumb into the muscle and tendons along the inside of the arm and armpit.
- Pull tension away from the bones by stretching or massaging between the striations of the muscle.
- Feel the lines and wiggle between them, loosening the nerves and lymph flow.
- Here you can switch from thumb to the four fingers.
- Breathe deeply into the armpit and shoulder, holding the breath in to expand, open and stretch from the inside and exhale to release.
- While you inhale, circle the arm and shoulder forward and back. Inhale up, exhale down.

UPPER ARMS + ELBOWS

Massaging the upper arms and elbows are vital for releasing emotional tension from the heart, lungs, and large and small intestines. By squeezing and massaging the elbows of either arm regularly you can relieve stress from the heart and help prevent tendonitis, arthritis and carpal tunnel syndrome.

- Continue massaging with the thumb down along the inside of the bone, gradually moving down the bicep towards the elbow.
- Massage the tendons along the bone, taking time to massage any tough or sensitive areas, scar tissue or tension.
- Once you are close to the elbow you should begin to feel a thin tendon just inside the elbow.
- Grip the lower arm bone from both sides and begin to pump the forearm.
- Pump the forearm and hand back and forth

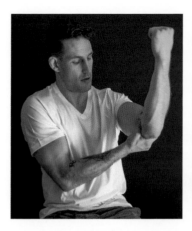 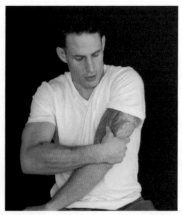

in an attempt to "loosen" the tendons, releasing pain in the elbow.

- Continue to squeeze and let go while loosening the elbow joint and bicep tendon, pumping the forearm then massaging the inside of the elbow, bicep and surrounding tissue and bones of the elbow joint.
- Hold and breathe into any injured or particularly sensitive places, let go and restore.
- Next, move your hand to the outside of the arm, gripping the tricep, squeezing the outside arm with the thumb.
- From the middle of the arm bone to the elbow, use the thumb to massage into the bone of the humerus while pumping the forearm.
- After massaging the upper arm, move down to the bottom of the elbow and use the thumb and index finger to lightly dig in and around the elbow.
- Squeeze the tip of the elbow with the thumb, index, and middle finger while you pump the arm, moving where you apply pressure, loosening tendons and releasing pain.

FOREARM + WRISTS

In reflexology, the wrists show a connection to the lower back and hips. Massaging and relaxing the wrists can not only help to release physical pain but can also ease emotional tension too. Use the following elbow technique to efficiently release and relax the tendons and ligaments of the wrist and forearm.

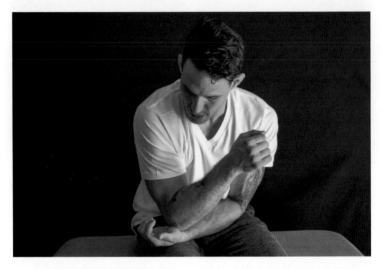

- Use your elbow to apply pressure into the forearm and wrist.
- Hold and breathe deeply as you feel the tension leaving through the fingertips.
- Inhale with the hand open, opening the palm and fingers.
- Exhale and release the hand, allowing the fingers to relax.
- Alternate between using your thumb and elbow to work down the forearm, relaxing the tension between the radius and ulnar bones (forearm bones), squeezing the forearm and

gradually moving down to the wrist.

- Press into the veins of the inner forearm and wrist using the elbow, clearing stale blood and energy, breathing deeply into any discomfort.
- After the right arm, switch and do the same to the left.

HANDS

Reflexology reveals that the hands are a map of the body. The wrists represent the hips, the center of the palm correlates to the kidneys, liver, spleen, small and large intestine, while the fingers represent the head and brain. Use the thumb, four fingers, and elbow to massage the hands regularly to build strength.

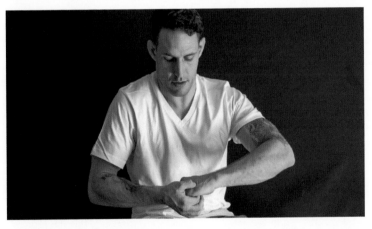

- Using the elbow, place pressure into the center of the palm.
- Massage the tendon and bones, back and forth, leading into the fingers.
- Press the elbow into the part of the palm near the thumb.
- Next, use the thumb and index finger to

squeeze the palm of the thumb. Hold on the nerve and breathe into it.

- Squeeze both sides of the entire hand (along the outside of the metacarpals of the pinky and index finger), move from the wrist and thumb up along the bones of the hand toward the fingers.
- After doing that on either hand, use the thumb and index finger to pinch/massage the webs between each finger as well as the top, bottom, and sides of each finger.
- Wiggle the bones open and apart.
- Be sure to squeeze all along the fingers, using the thumb to dig into the tissue between joints.
- Now, wiggle each joint side to side, releasing pressure from the joints of the three phalanges (finger bones).
- Pull the tip of each finger rapidly snapping and releasing energy from the ends of the nerves. This will help relieve the nervous system as each finger connects to a particular meridian.
- Shake out the hands and lightly pound or hit them onto the thighs.

CHEST + RIBCAGE

If the chest and ribcage become tight, it makes it more difficult for the lungs to breathe fully. When the lungs are not able to take a full breath, this makes the heart and blood have to work harder with less oxygen. By massaging the chest and muscles of the rib cage you can ease the heart and restore the respiratory system.

- Feeling down into the chest, use the index

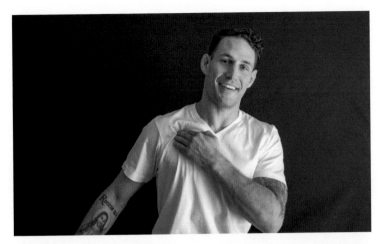

finger and middle finger together to push into the space just under and along the clavicle.

- Breathe deeply into the chest, expanding the lungs and rib cage as you press in between the ribs, shoulders, and chest.
- Next, move to the sides of the rib cage and with your thumbs, press in between the ribs, as you lean from side to side.
- It may also feel good to make two fists and squeeze the ribs as you exhale, stretching the ribs and compressing the lungs.

HEART + THYMUS

Emotion: Impatience / Love + Compassion
Color: Red • Sound: "HAAAA"

The thymus gland is responsible for making white blood cells which are the main defenders against bacteria and illness in the body. This gland is located in the very middle of the chest behind the sternum, to the right of the heart. Massaging the thymus gland regularly will help strengthen white blood cells and the entire immune system.

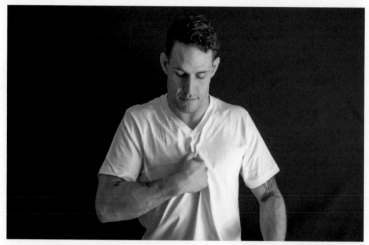

- With a fist, massage with your knuckles (shaking or swirling motion) into the bony area of the middle of the chest. Inhale and hold while you lean back slightly.
- Press the four fingers into the middle of the chest where the ribs connect, massaging away from the bone.
- Next, interlace the fingers together placing the hands high on the chest with pressure.
- Squeeze both elbows to the sides of your ribs.
- Inhale deeply and hold while looking up and back.
- Stretch your neck while slowly swaying the body from side to side.
- Exhale and come back to a relaxed neutral position.

SOLAR (CELIAC) PLEXUS

The solar plexus is the space below the rib-cage 1-2 inches above the navel or belly button. Located at the center of the body, it can be a sensitive area for some because it is the intersection of all the nerves in the abdomen.

Tension builds from the small intestine and heart, the liver and gallbladder, and the stomach, spleen, and pancreas, all meeting here in the middle to communicate through the spine. Massaging here regularly will help soften emotions throughout the entire body.

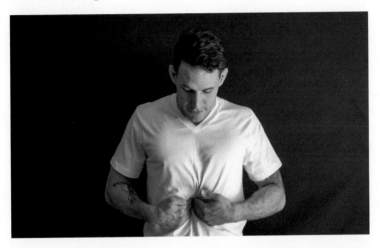

- With the index finger and middle finger of both hands, begin adding force, circling, and massaging.
- If sensitive...inhale and hold pressure, exhaling with an "HAAAA" sound.
- Focus on releasing feelings of resentment, grief, or impatience through the breath and out of the pores.
- Follow with an inhale of patience, love, and compassion.

SMALL INTESTINE

Emotion: Impatience / Love + Compassion
Color: Red • Sound: "HAAAA"

Just below the solar plexus directly under and

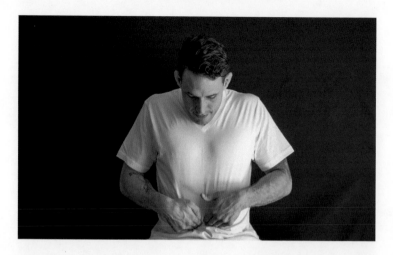

around the navel lies the small intestine. The small intestine is the center of digestion and connected to the heart along the aorta and heart meridian. The emotions of the stomach influence the small intestine as it is next in line in the digestion process.

- Use the four fingers of both hands and put pressure on either side of the navel.
- While applying pressure and massage, begin to shake the organ to loosen tension.
- You may potentially feel sharp pains and if so, hold at the point of pain, inhale, smile and center your mind on the feeling of gratitude.
- Use the feeling of appreciation to heal the heart and small intestine and replace negative stress with good intention exhaling with the heart sound "HAAAA."

LIVER + GALLBLADDER
Emotion: Anger + Frustration / Kindness + Generosity
Color: Green • Sound: "SHHH"
To the right of the solar plexus are the liver and

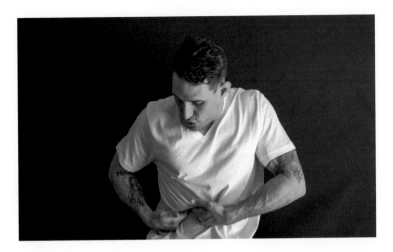

gallbladder. Held emotions of anger and frustration can contribute to the hardening of the liver and affect the gall bladder. By practicing feelings of kindness and generosity, this will help to soften the liver and surrounding organs.

- Start by replacing any negative thoughts with feelings of kindness and generosity.
- Slightly lean to the left and inhale to expand the right side rib cage where the liver is.
- Then exhale 6-9 seconds with a "SHHH" sound folding to the right, compressing the liver and gallbladder.
- Hold the exhale as long as you feel comfortable, relaxing and releasing tension.
- Using the four fingers on or under the ribs of the right side, pump the liver 3-9 times.
- Once you've finished pumping the liver, place your palms over the right ribs and feel a warm sensation of peace and kindness wash over you, softening the liver and gallbladder.

STOMACH + SPLEEN + PANCREAS
Emotion: Worry + Anxiety / Openness + Trust
Color: Yellow • Sound: "WHOOO"

Moving to the left side of the abdomen just under the ribcage is your stomach, spleen, and pancreas. Massaging this area can help to relieve built up anxiety, worry, and mistrust. Not only will worries and anxious energy seem to fall away the more you consciously practice openness and trust, but massaging and clearing these negative emotions will help to strengthen the tissue and improve the overall health of these organs.

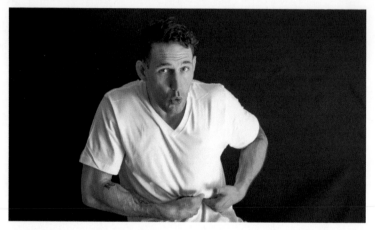

- Place both palms on the left side of your ribs.
- Inhale deeply, opening up the left side of the ribs by leaning to your right.
- Hold the inhale to expand and stretch the stomach and surrounding tissue and tendons.
- Folding to your left, exhale with a "WHOO" sound and with your four fingers, dig under the left ribs, massaging into the stomach and spleen.

- Inhale with a smile, feeling emotions of fairness, openness, and trust through the nose while pulling up with the pelvic floor.
- Using the four fingers on or under the ribs on the left side, pump the stomach 3-9 times.
- Once you've finished pumping the stomach, spleen and left side, place your palms over the left ribs and feel a warm sensation of trust and confidence washing over and softening the left side.

LUNGS
Emotion: Grief + Sadness / Strength + Courage
Color: White • Sound: "SSSSS"

The lungs can hold emotions of sadness and grief which in some cases make it hard to breathe properly, experiencing symptoms of shallow breathing, asthma, and low energy levels. When the shoulders fold forward for whatever reason (poor posture, heartaches, emotions, habits, etc.), this can make it difficult for the lungs to fully open.

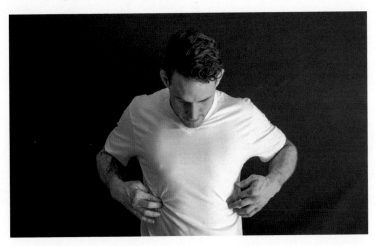

The upper lung points are at the chest and front shoulders, while the lower lung points are on either side of the ribcage at the lower floating ribs, just above the hips.

- Massage into the upper chest just below the shoulder with light circles using the four fingers or knuckles.
- Press into the side of the ribs with the thumbs, massaging lightly to ease and relax any and each pain point found.
- Because the lungs hold grief and sadness, exhaling and releasing these emotions with intention will allow for deeper, stronger breaths.
- Inhale the emotions of strength, courage, and righteousness.
- Exhale with an "SSSSS" sound as you release.

LARGE INTESTINE

Emotion: Grief + Sadness / Strength + Courage
Color: White • Sound: "SSSSS"

The large intestine wraps around the exterior of the small intestine starting at the lower right side of the belly, just above the hip bone. Continuing up the right side of the abdomen is the ascending colon, turning at the liver (right ribs), running along the top of the small intestine towards the spleen (left ribs). It then continues down the descending colon to the sigmoid colon at the left hip.

By massaging the tissue of the large intestine regularly you can strengthen the muscle and tissue, speeding up digestion, absorption and elimination, effectively giving you more energy, and slimming the waist and belly.

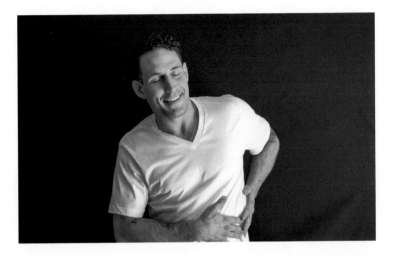

- Lightly use both the palms and fingers to rub the belly clockwise, following the natural flow of the large intestine. This will help to move excess waste and energy through the organ to aid in digestion and elimination.
- Next, use the four fingers to massage the bottom right corner of the belly, just above the hip bone.
- With a scooping motion dig into the lower belly, pulling tension away from the hip bone.
- Don't be afraid to dig deep, a lot of tension sits in the hips affecting the large intestine and bladder.
- After massaging the lower belly, move upward along the right side of the abdomen, massaging into the obliques up the right side.
- Follow up the ascending colon, moving any knots you feel upward.
- Once at the top near the liver and ribs, circle clockwise inward and counterclockwise outward to release tension. Do this 3-9 times while inhaling into the lower right side.

- Move across to the left of the abdomen just below the spleen and stomach.
- Once you are at the top left corner of the abdomen, just under the ribs, gently circle inward and outward 3-9 times, then continue down the descending colon to the left hip.
- The end of the large intestine seems to be a sensitive grief point for a majority of people who have a hard time letting go of past trauma. Sadness and grief can get stuck at the sigmoid colon, being the final "let go" point physically and energetically.
- Release negative energy, pain, and any blockages from the lower-left corner of the abdomen by using the four fingers to dig away tension from the hip bone and pelvic floor.
- Be sure to hold pressure and dig deep enough into the space between the navel and left hip. Feel for hard spots to massage and breathe into them. You may also use a baseball or medicine ball to lie on and get a deeper pressure.
- Relax any knots and tensions, exhaling with the lung and large intestine sound "SSSSS", inhaling strength, courage, and righteousness, feeling a sense of accomplishment and strength through practice.

To see each exercise in detail on video, please visit **Academy.NewLifeCNT.com** *and watch the course.*

PART 3

LOWER BODY

"Jing" is *"the energy produced by the earth and sexual organs with which we can recharge, stimulate and rejuvenate ourselves."* It is the vitality that we use to bring forth new life and ensure good health in our older years. When we lose too much of this *Jing* energy, we may become devitalized and can show signs of premature aging.

The kidneys are our great reservoir of *Jing* energy and are associated with longevity, vitality, sexual energy and our creative powers.

To lead a long and healthy life, one must accumulate an abundance of *Jing* to recharge the kidneys and avoid losing this vital energy. *Jing* governs the strength of our structural frame, hair, nails, healing powers, sexual functions and reproductive potential, youthfulness and the ability to handle stress, adversity, and overwork.

While massaging, concentrate on inhaling and pulling up on the pelvic floor to guide this energy up the spine and replenish the kidneys, surrounding organs, and brain, training your awareness and internal functions.

COMMON LOWER BODY ISSUES

Common lower body issues include but are not

limited to; lower back pain, herniations, hemorrhages, hip pain, sciatic pain, digestion issues, abdominal pains, cramps, lower energy, low testosterone, prostate issues, erectile dysfunction, ovary pain, bladder pains, tight psoas, knee pains, plantar fascitis, and restless leg syndrome. Regular self-massage will ease pain from multiple sources, effectively changing the subconscious patterning of dysfunction.

BLADDER
Emotion: Fear / Peace + Security
Color: Dark Blue • Sound: "CHOOO"

The bladder is located 1-2 inches below the navel or belly button, just above the pelvic bone. Holding and filtering not only the liquid waste of our body but our emotional waste as well. A soft healthy bladder allows for proper filtration of emotions.

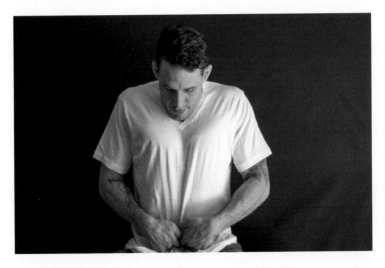

- Using the four fingers of both hands, massage in a scooping motion, pulling the bladder up and away from the pelvic bone. This will help strengthen the tissue of the bladder and lower ab area.

- You may also feel the need to go to the bathroom but this is not only due to liquids but a large amount of unrefined energy stored in the bladder as well.
- While massaging, visualize this energy like steam moving up the body to help nourish the kidneys and other organs.
- The point just below the navel is called the lower **Dāntián** (or **tan t'ien**) and is believed to be an energy storehouse of the body where both Yin (water from the earth) and Yang (fire from the heavens) meet.
- Imagine circulating both hot and cold energies in the lower *Dāntián* to create warm energy, combining cold yin with hot yang.
- Rub your palms in small circles over the bladder clockwise and counterclockwise 3-9 times, feeling the warmth relaxing and soothing the organ.

KIDNEYS

Emotion: Fear / Peace + Security
Color: Dark Blue • Sound: "CHOOO"

After working on the bladder, move your hands around to the middle of your back on either side of the spine where you'll find both kidneys between the fourth and fifth ribs.

The right kidney tends to be lower than the left because the liver, being somewhat large, pushes the right kidney downward. This is another reason to detox and clear the liver so that it doesn't put added stress on the right kidney.

The kidneys are powerful batteries of Jing energy. The adrenal glands which control the output of adrenaline are above the kidneys and just under the heart. These important glands must be nourished and treated with special care.

Massaging the kidneys, bladder, and sexual organs regularly to soothe and restore the adrenal glands can help to strengthen the will and overall energy of a person, replenishing the nervous system and all functions of the body and brain.

By massaging into the kidneys and bladder daily, it's been found to help eliminate feelings of fear, allowing for more peace, calmness, and clarity.

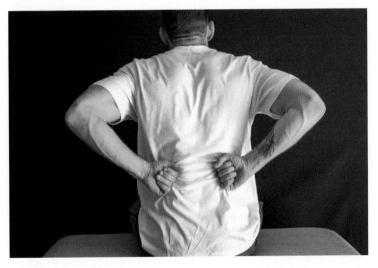

- Reach around the back and make two fists. Using the knuckles of the index finger, dig into the muscle on either side of the spine.
- Next, gently hit, knock or pound the lower back and ribs with the back of both fists. This will vibrate and help clear tension away before massaging deeper.

- Again, with the index knuckle of the fist, place pressure firmly, shaking, circling and holding at any place that feels sensitive.
- Inhale into the kidneys and lower back, feeling the ribs of the back expand.
- Exhale 3-9 seconds with a hollowed out "CHOOO" sound pulling the belly in and folding to the left, compressing the left kidney.
- Inhale emotions of peace, gentleness, and faith as you expand the back ribs, nourishing the left side, rubbing your palms gently on the back left side to feel a warm calming sensation.
- Exhale and rest before moving to the right side and turning your attention to the right kidney.
- Inhale to expand the back and right side of the ribcage.
- Exhale 3-9 seconds with a "CHOOO" sound, pulling the belly in and bending to the right.
- Hold the exhale out as long as you can then inhale emotions of peace, gentleness, and faith, pulling up the muscles of the pelvic floor.
- Exhale with the kidney sound, relaxing the sexual organs, bladder, and pelvic floor.
- To finish massaging the kidneys, place your palms over both kidneys on the back and visualize breathing into your palms and kidneys on either side.
- Feel the warmth gather into the lower back and sense a calm gentle peace washing over you.

SACRUM

Moving down the spine to the very bottom is the sacrum or "tailbone." The sacrum is located just below the lumbar or lower spine and is a combination of 3-5 smaller bones that need to be somewhat flexible and open for proper flow of spinal fluid.

The sacrum is said to be the control board of the body, because it is at the center of the skeletal system. The bones make blood from the nervous system and it's various responses and emotional state, producing adaptogens for the body to defend itself against oncoming attacks. Hitting and massaging the sacrum can build up the nervous system, effectively strengthening the entire body.

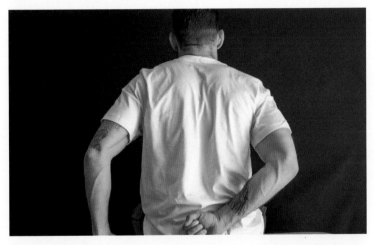

- Use the back of the fist to hit the bones of the sacrum and loosen tension from the surrounding tissue and nerves.
- Breathe into the sacrum, imagining the breath going through eight holes of this bone, opening the nerve and energy channels (this may take time to imagine and feel the sacrum open, as the sacrum tends to

get very tight and stiff over time if never opened intentionally).

- Use the index finger, knuckle, and thumbs to massage around the sacrum following along the iliac crest (hip bones) on either side.

HIPS

The hips can carry a variety of emotions relating to fear and sadness. The kidney meridians located along the back of the legs into the sacrum and spine, and bladder and large intestine sitting within the bowl of the pelvis, the sciatic nerve and surrounding muscles and tendons (including the IT band) can all become tight and rigged from stress, causing pain and weakness. This is most commonly caused by long hours of sitting, intense workouts, and or added pressure from either being overweight or pregnant. By simply massaging the hip bones and sciatic nerve regularly with the thumbs and knuckles you can relieve physical pain and with continual practice, ease negative emotions.

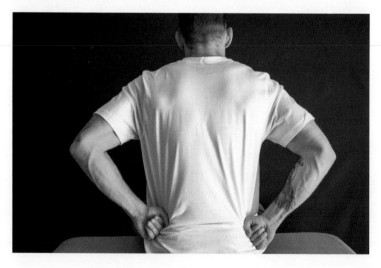

- Use your thumbs on either side and massage into the hip bone and surrounding muscle, feeling for sensitivity.
- In addition to using your thumbs, make a fist and use the index knuckles to dig into the underside of either hip bone.
- Just below the hip bone you'll find the sciatic nerve which can be a sensitive spot. Hold and breathe deep into the belly while expanding the hips.

SEXUAL ORGANS

Emotion: Fear / Peace + Security
Color: Dark Blue • Sound: "CHOOO"

Massaging the sexual organs are different for men and women. As men massage the testicles and bladder, women massage the ovaries, uterus, bladder, and breasts.

Women

Massaging the ovaries and breasts are the most important areas for overall energy, sexual organ and kidney health. Breasts are connected to the uterus, which is connected to the ovaries, and the ovaries are connected to the bladder and kidneys. The ovaries are located on either side of the belly button, 2-3 inches down between both A.S.I.S (front hip bones).

This massage technique is beneficial for all women, at any age or stage of life.

- Begin massaging by using the index and middle fingers to put pressure on the front hips and ovaries.
- With gentle pressure, make small circles inward and outward 3-9 times both clockwise and counterclockwise.

- Create a warm peaceful energy here by smiling then inhaling, pulling energy upwards to nourish the kidneys and adrenal glands.
- To massage the breasts, use the palms of the hands to make small outward circles around the nipples into larger circles cycling energy out and down into the ovaries.
- Do this 3-9 times, stimulating and creating energy to nourish the ovaries. After infusing energy into the ovaries, bring Chi back up into the kidneys to nourish the rest of the body by focusing on the warm sensations.
- Also, pinching and stimulating the nipples helps to contract the uterus. This can be especially beneficial after pregnancy to bring the uterus back to its normal size. This is also why a child needs to nurse from its mother's breast (for the child, and for the mother).

Men

Sexual tension can cause energy blockages within the pelvic area (i.e. prostate, scrotum, and penis) including mental, physical and emotional reactions, pains, aches, and inabilities.

Massaging the testicles and guiding this energy upward is important for balancing sexual energy, increasing testosterone levels, preventing prostate issues, and strengthening sexual functions.

- When massaging the male genitals, begin by pressing the index and middle finger into the *perineum* area between the anus and genitals, relaxing the lower pelvic floor. Tensions may originally be caused by either too much or a lack of sexual stimulation, sitting for long periods, and stress held in the groin; more commonly connected to the emotion of fear.

- After clearing tension from this area between the anus and groin, begin to lightly squeeze each testicle one at a time. You should be able to feel a small cord coming from the end of the testicle, called the *spermatic cord.* Due to stress over time this cord builds small clumps of tissue in and around where sperm is made and sent out.
- You may feel some pain in the belly and kidneys while clearing this small knotted area as it goes up into the bladder and kidneys. Inhale into this feeling, pulling energy up into the kidneys and exhale to relax the pelvic floor completely. The left testicle is connected to the left kidney and the right testicle is connected to the right kidney.
- While squeezing the spermatic cord and testicle, massage away the pain by exhaling with a hollowed-out "CHOOO" sound, contracting the anus, perineum, and genital muscles to feel energy rising up the spine.
- Breathe deeply into the belly to fill the scrotum and pelvic floor. With each inhale lightly contract these lower muscles pulling up the warm energy produced into the kidneys and adrenal glands, clearing and nourishing energy and health. Exhale and relax.
- Take 3-9 full breaths here, feeling a sense of peace, calm, and gentleness wash over you.

THIGHS

The femur bones are one of the biggest bones in the body. The bones, more specifically the bone marrow, make all of the blood within the body. When stress is a common part of some-one's day, the quality and health of the blood produced are affected.

When the body becomes overly stressed ac-companied by long hours of sitting knees and poor posture, energy gets blocked and locked in the thighs. When seated for too long, the proper flow of digestion is affected physically and ener-getically. Over time, the body has trouble elimi-nating physical and emotional waste.

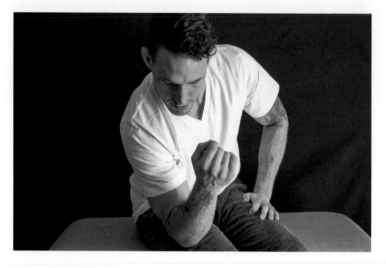

- To release this blockage use the elbows to press into the thigh bones starting from the top hip flexors.
- Feel for a large tendon and just inside of it you will feel the femoral arteries.
- Continue massaging in half circles moving down the inner thigh, stretching and open-ing muscles along the groin and thighs on either leg.
- After clearing the inner thighs and groin,

follow around to the outside of the thighs, along the TFL or outer thighs. You may also like to try lying on a tennis ball or foam roller for added pressure.

- Be sure to take time massaging the thighs and know that it will take multiple sittings to release years of unconscious tension.

KNEES

Massaging the knees regularly will help to clear old Chi, fascia and blood out of the joints, tendons and tissue, supporting cells to reproduce in a stronger and healthier way. Slapping and massaging, squeezing, and breathing helps to break down built-up stress, tension, and pressure behind the knees, increasing circulation and ease.

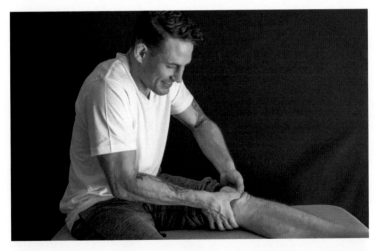

- Begin by slapping/patting the front and back of the knees. This can be done every morning to clear away stagnant Chi and bring new blood and warmth into the knees.
- Use the index fingers and thumbs around the top of the knees and thighs. Begin by pressing

the index fingers into the soft tissue under and around the patella (kneecap).

- Feeling for tightness, place firm pressure into any hard tissue. Try to soften and make the patella flexible in all directions.
- Next, with the palms, rub, squeeze and massage tension down into the shin warming the knees with new blood.
- Finally, squeeze the thumbs and index fingers into the sides of the knee, digging into the joints behind and under the kneecap, making sure the kneecap is flexible in all directions.

ANKLE

Energetically, the ankles are our support system between the knees and the feet. As the kidney meridians are located along the legs, emotions of fear and instability can affect the strength of the bones and tendons, which in turn weaken the ankles leading to possible injury. By massaging the ankles with both hands and elbows periodically, you can help to realign and strengthen the bones and tendons.

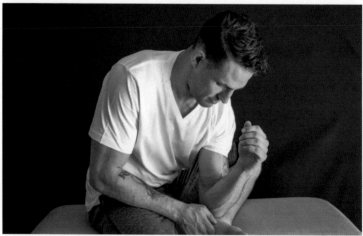

The Achilles tendon, which runs up the back of the leg from the heel to the knee, can affect both the feet and the knee. Massaging and elongating this tendon helps to prevent issues such as plantar fasciitis, knee injuries and chronic pain.

- Massage down into the shins, pulling muscle and tissue away from the shin bones, squeezing the calves with the thumbs and four fingers, progressing down into the ankles, pushing the excess tension down into the earth.
- Squeeze the ankles firmly, massaging half-circles into the front ankles on either side.
- Use the elbow to put pressure into the back of the ankle, separating the Achilles from the heel. This will help to strengthen the tendon.
- Use the thumbs to massage and relax into the calves.
- Follow with the elbow all along the whole Achilles from the calves to the heel.

FEET

The kidney meridians start from the feet. This means that the energy connecting from the earth to the adrenal glands should be in communication. When there are blockages or knots along these connections negative emotions begin to surface. By massaging tension from the feet you can release emotions of fear and shame held in the foundation of your body, restoring peace and a gentle nature.

- Massage the Achilles tendon with the thumbs and bridge of the index finger, following the ankle and pressing firmly into the base of the foot, squeezing the heel.
- Next, firmly hit the base of the heel with the

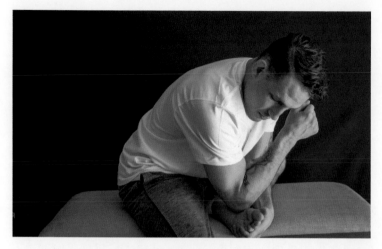

front knuckles of the four fingers in a half fist position. Knocking on the bones all over the foot then going up into the leg.

- Place both hands on one foot, massaging the inner arch.
- Then place the foot over the other knee if comfortable, and press both thumbs into the muscle of the inner foot, massaging between the ball of the foot and heel.
- Using an elbow may be more effective as well.
- Press, hold, and massage in small circles and side to side or up and down motions until all soreness or tenderness goes away (you will need to do this more than once, so take your time and breathe deeply into the feet and smile).
- Press on the ball of the foot massaging be-tween the joints of the foot leading into the toes.
- Squeeze the toes, pulling/snapping energy off of them.
- Place the fingers between the web of each

of the toes with the index finger and thumb around the big toe.

- Stretch the toes and open them to allow for more blood and Chi.
- Making space between the toes helps with circulation, clarity, and balance.
- A major point on the bottom of the foot is the (K1) kidney point or "bubbling spring." It is located directly between the big toe and second toe on the ball of the foot. You can very easily activate this point by standing on your toes while inhaling. Imagining the Earth's restorative Yin energy rising through the feet up into the pelvis, kidneys, and adrenal glands for more energy.
- Once on your toes, fall back onto your heels into the earth and feel the vibration and relaxation throughout the entire body.

*To see each exercise in detail on video, please visit **Academy.NewLifeCNT.com** and watch the course.*

THIS PAGE IS
INTENTIONALLY LEFT BLANK

PART 4

CONCLUSION

PART 4
CONCLUSION

Emotion is energy in motion. When we hold onto negative emotions, it becomes trapped in our body at deep levels. The countless hours of studying the concepts and practices of **Qigong**, meditations, and massage have led to the experiences that created this book. If I had not learned Chi Nei Tsang and the practices found in this book, I would have continued to suffer from depression, anxiety, grief, frustration, and fear. Learning these spiritual arts and sciences has been one of the most healing and rewarding works I have yet to accomplish.

My hope in writing this guidebook is that it will inspire self-healing and internal development in everyone who reads it. We all have the power to change our perception and take the proper steps to improve and gain power over our ailments and issues.

If you enjoyed this book and would like to continue your study of Chi Nei Tsang, as well as learn from me, you can follow me online and take the course on *Self-Massage Secrets* (and other upcoming courses) at *Academy.NewLifeCNT.com*.

We must follow the five elements and keep each organ and emotion in check. Only then will we experience every blessing in our life. Helping, healing, and holding in positive vibration. Attracting and receiving that which we put out. Love, trust, courage, peace, kindness...energy in motion.

Follow your heart and listen to the voice of life, take faith into your future, and live joyously. May healing love and peace be with you.

ABOUT THE AUTHOR

Niko Carrafield is a lifelong student of Qigong, Yoga, Martial arts and all things health and wellness. He first discovered Tai Chi and Qigong when he was 17, and learned Tai Chi from Dr. Lu and Master Yang in Irvine, CA, and online study of Qigong Internal Meditations from Master Mantak Chia.

Niko received his certification at the Universal Healing Tao Center in Chiang Mai, Thailand. Through the Tao, we learn that trapped emotions, trauma, and memories held in the subconcious mind and body contribute to disease and Chi Nei Tsang is a process to eliminate them.

Now certified in Chi Nei Tsang 1 & 2, Reiki, Cosmic Healing, and Yoga, Niko found peace in massaging the body and using the breath to transform consciousness from negative to positive emotions. He has personally transformed his emotional imbalances (such as anger, grief and anxiety along with issues of tonsilitis, strep, tinnitus and skin disorders) into a stronger, well-balanced immune system and a more relaxed and restored state of emotions.

Through Chi Nei Tsang and the discovery of yoga and Qigong practices, self-massage, mantras, and meditations, Niko has been able to change his attitude about how healing takes place to let go of past beliefs and adopt a new mindset of hope, health, and happiness. His one true goal in writing this book is to pass on this knowledge and ability to others so they can benefit and find healing as well.

ACKNOWLEDGEMENTS

The information provided in this book was originally introduced and discovered through the study and teachings of Qigong, Chi Nei Tsang, Reflexology, Acupressure, Cosmic Healing, and Reiki.

I'd like to thank Master Mantak Chia, at the Universal Healing Tao Center located in Chiang Mai, Thailand for his vast knowledge and teachings of QiGong and Chi Nei Tsang.

For more information on the use and practice of Chi Nei Tsang, QiGong, Acupressure and Reiki, visit **NewLifeCNT.com**.